OXFORD MEDICAL PUBLICATIONS

Cervical Screening

PRACTICAL GUIDES FOR GENERAL PRACTICE

Editorial Board

J. A. Muir Gray, Community Physician,
Oxfordshire Health Authority.
Ann McPherson, General Practitioner, Oxford.
Michael Bull, GP Tutor, Oxford.
John Tasker, GP Tutor, North Oxfordshire.

Cervical Screening

SECOND EDITION

Practical Guides for General Practice 14

by
JOAN AUSTOKER
Director, C.R.C. Primary Care Education Group, Oxford

ANN McPHERSON
General Practitioner, Oxford

This guide has been produced in association with the Cancer Research Campaign and the Imperial Cancer Research Fund

Oxford   New York   Tokyo
OXFORD UNIVERSITY PRESS
1992

Oxford University Press, Walton Street, Oxford OX2 6DP

Oxford New York Toronto
Delhi Bombay Calcutta Madras Karachi
Petaling Jaya Singapore Hong Kong Tokyo
Nairobi Dar es Salaam Cape Town
Melbourne Auckland

and associated companies in
Berlin Ibadan

Oxford is a trade mark of Oxford University Press

Published in the United States
by Oxford University Press, New York

A catalogue record for this book is available from the British Library

Library of Congress Cataloging in Publication Data
Austoker, Joan.
Cervical screening/by Joan Austoker, Ann McPherson.—2nd ed.
(Oxford medical publications)
Includes bibliographical references and index.
1. Cervix uteri—Cancer—Cytodiagnosis—Handbooks, manuals, etc.
2. Medical screening—Handbooks, manuals, etc. I. McPherson, Ann.
Cervical screening. II. Title. III. Series. IV. Series: Oxford
medical publications.
[DNLM: 1. Cervix Dysplasia—prevention & control. 2. Cervix
Neoplasms—prevention & control. 3. Mass Screening.
W1 PR141NK no. 14/WP480 A938c]
RC280.U8A89 1991   362.1'9699466—dc20   91-31833
ISBN 0–19–262170–X (pbk.)

Typeset by Cotswold Typesetting Limited, Cheltenham
Printed in Great Britain by
Dotesios Ltd, Trowbridge, Wilts

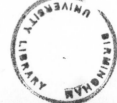

Preface

Cervical screening: a practical guide was first published in 1985. At that time cervical screening in the UK was operating in a fairly haphazard way. The idea of the first booklet was to offer a practical yet detailed and universally applicable approach to help primary care team-members—doctors, nurses, receptionists, and practice managers—set up and develop effective cervical screening programmes.

Since that time major changes have occurred in the area of cervical screening. The introduction in 1988 of a systematic call and recall system and the setting up of an NHS Cervical Screening Programme National Co-ordinating Network has brought a greater sense of coherence. A more consistent and uniform approach is being formulated for deciding who should be screened and how often, for classifying smears according to the degree of nuclear abnormality, for standardizing terminology, for interpreting results and following up abnormalities, and for evaluating the programme. Steps are being taken nationally by Health Authorities to improve the effectiveness of local programmes.

Primary care remains central to the success of the programme. The vast majority of smears will be taken in general practice. GPs will also be responsible for issuing results, ensuring adequate follow-up, and providing counselling and support where appropriate. The 1990 GP contract has set targets upon which payment for cervical screening depends.

Many problems still exist. Key amongst these is the question of coverage, an area in which primary care can exert a major influence. At present screening resources are being inappropriately concentrated on the younger, lower-risk groups. More than half the smears are being taken from women under the age of 35, among whom only 16 per cent of cases of invasive cancer occur. To be most effective screening must concentrate on a wide age-range, with every effort being made to reach those at relatively higher risk of developing invasive cancer, namely older women of lower social classes.

Ultimately there is a need for a cheaper and more specific test. Debates on cost-effectiveness and efficacy have a place in any deliberation; but measuring effectiveness in human, social, and economic terms is far from straightforward or precise, and involves value judgements. For the present we must work with what is currently available and endeavour to make the cervical screening programme operate more efficiently than it has in the past. To ensure that this is the case we will need to monitor and evaluate the outcomes.

This booklet aims to provide practices with a practical approach to cervical screening. It covers a wide range of topics, from facts on the disease and advice on running an effective call–recall system to recommendations on follow-up procedures and a discussion on the controversies and unresolved areas which still exist. We hope you find it useful.

Oxford   J. A.
July 1991   A. M.

Acknowledgements

We owe a great debt of gratitude to many people who have helped us in the course of preparing this book. Muir Gray and members of the NHS Cervical Screening Programme National Co-ordinating Network have been a constant source of help and advice. Ian Duncan has provided invaluable advice and constructive criticism on numerous occasions. This has done much to ensure the accuracy of the information in the book. Many others have also commented at length on various drafts of the book. In particular we would like to thank Gary Cook, Winifred Gray, Amanda Herbert, Elizabeth Hudson, John Humphreys, Elizabeth MacKenzie, Jackie Maxmin, Rachel Miller, John Modle, Simon Plint, Angela Raffle, Jon Rogers, Sam Rowlands, Peter Sasieni. We remain responsible for any errors of fact or interpretation in the text.

The production of this book and its distribution to general practices throughout the UK would not have been possible without the generous support of the Cancer Research Campaign and Imperial Cancer Research Fund.

Contents

1 The guidelines

Who should be screened?

All women aged 20–64 who are or ever have been sexually active.

When should screening stop?

Age 65 is suggested. However, women aged 65 and over should be encouraged to have a smear if they have not previously been screened.

How often should smears be taken?

Every 3 to 5 years.

The Department of Health recommends that a smear should be taken 'at least every 5 years' (DHSS 1988). At present 29 per cent of District Health Authorities (DHAs) operate a 5-year recall, 25 per cent a 3-year recall. The remainder operate a mixture of 3- and 5-year recalls according to age (Elkind et al. 1990).

29% 5
25% 3
rest 5/3 according to age

2   Cervical cancer: the facts

Incidence

In the UK during 1985 (the latest year for which figures are available, 4496 new cases of invasive cervical cancer were registered (see Fig. 1). This makes it the eighth most common cancer in women, with an incidence rate of 158 new cases per million population. Eighty-four per cent of new cases of invasive cancer occurred in women aged 35 and over. About 9000 women were registered with pre-malignant conditions (see Fig. 2). The vast majority (87 per cent) of *in situ* cases were registered in younger women under the ages of 45 years, which may be a reflection of the higher prevalence of screening among younger women (see pp. 8–11).

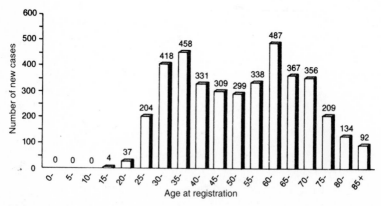

Fig. 1. Invasive cancer of the cervix—new cases registered, England and Wales 1985. (Source: CRC Factsheet 12, 1990.)

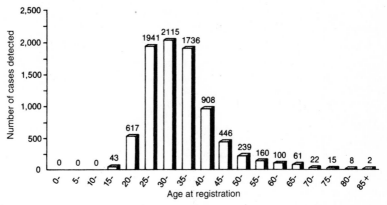

Fig. 2. Carcinoma *in situ* of the cervix: new cases registered, England and Wales 1985. (From 1984 onwards registrations of *in situ* patients have included those with a mention of cervical intra-epithelial neoplasia grade 3 (CIN3).) (Source: CRC Factsheet 12, 1990.)

The cohort effect ᴵ⁹²⁹

Women born in the five years around 1921 have higher rates of invasive carcinoma of the cervix and higher mortality rates throughout their lives than for previous birth cohorts this century. For subsequent birth cohorts the rates are lower until 1941. From the 1941 birth cohort onwards the cohort incidence and mortality rates have increased progressively. Women born around 1951 have twice the risk of dying from cervical cancer than women born in 1941. The progressively higher incidence and mortality rates for more recent cohorts fits the theory that cervical cancer could be a sexually transmitted disease whose spread has been facilitated by freer sexual relationships.

4 Cervical screening

Survival

The national five-year relative survival rate for all women treated for invasive cervical cancer in 1981 in England and Wales was 57 per cent. However survival after diagnosis and treatment is directly related to stage at the time of diagnosis (see Table 1). The survival is much higher in women who are diagnosed and treated at an early stage. The marked difference in survival prognosis for different stages provides an incentive to screen women routinely.

Table 1. Stage and prognosis

Stage	Description	5-year survival rate %
	Precancerous lesions	99–100
I	Cancer confined to the cervix	79
II	Cancer has spread beyond the cervix but not on to the pelvic wall	47
III	Cancer has spread on to the pelvic wall	22
IV	Cancer has spread more widely	7
All stages		57

Source: CRC Factsheet 12.

International variation

Worldwide, cancer of the cervix is the second most common female cancer, with some 460 000 cases occurring every year; 77 per cent of these occur in the developing world. In the developing countries it is the commonest female cancer, with very high incidence rates being recorded in China, Latin America, and the Caribbean.

An analysis of mortality in a large number of countries

throughout the world confirms that cervical cancer mortality is declining in many parts of the developed world; but in several countries, including Scotland, England, and Wales, although the 'all ages' rates are decreasing, in younger women mortality is increasing.

Risk factors

Factors related to risk, either directly or indirectly, include:

- Sexual behaviour
- Sexual transmission
- Parity, and age at first pregnancy
- Method of contraception
- Occupation and social class
- Heavy smoking
- A history of dyskaryosis

Primary prevention

At present, the exact cause of cervical cancer is not known. Unfortunately, therefore, definitive advice on primary prevention is not possible. Moreover, from what we do know of its causes, primary prevention may not be socially acceptable. However, women should have enough information of possible causes to allow decisions to be made which may help in primary prevention.

- In some way sex is involved, and women with many partners, or whose partners have many partners, are more at risk.

- Parity and age at first pregnancy: virgin women have the lowest risk and women having a late first pregnancy have a lower relative risk than those with an early pregnancy.

An increased number of pregnancies increases the risk of cervical abnormalities; but this may be due to associated sexual behaviour such as age at first intercourse and number of partners.

- The method of contraception may be important. Barrier methods are protective, and long-term use of the pill may increase the risk.

- The present thinking is that certain strains of the papilloma or wart virus may be involved, although this has not been proved with any degree of certainty. Women should be advised about the possible risks of having intercourse with a man with penile warts unless he is using a condom.

- Mortality statistics for cervical cancer show a steep reverse social-class gradient, with the disease being three times as common in social class 5 as in the professional classes. Primary prevention is obviously not feasible on the grounds of social class. What is important is for screening to reach those in lower social classes who are at relatively higher risk of developing invasive cervical cancer (see p. 11).

- Heavy smoking (more than 20 cigarettes a day) has emerged as a risk factor for cervical cancer. Women should be advised of the benefits of giving up or reducing smoking—this would not only reduce the risk of cervical cancer but of lung cancer and coronary heart disease.

> *Remember when giving advice about primary prevention this should be non-judgemental and avoid any sense of victim-blaming.*

3 Cervical screening: the facts

Organized screening programmes have been in operation in parts of Europe and North America for well over 20 years. Despite the success of cervical screening in some of the Nordic countries and elsewhere, for example British Columbia and the NE of Scotland, there is not yet a consensus on how screening should be organized. In Britain, where screening has been operating since 1964, it is hard to detect any substantial effect of screening, although detailed analyses of trends suggest that any observed increases in incidence of and mortality from invasive cervical cancer might have been much greater in the absence of screening.

Screening in the Nordic countries

There are no randomized controlled trials demonstrating the effectiveness of cervical screening in reducing mortality. The evidence for its benefit is derived mainly from the comparison of trends in incidence and mortality in those countries in which there is well organized screening and those countries which, at least in the past, have not had well-organized screening, the United Kingdom falling into the latter category.

The Nordic countries have adopted very different policies towards cervical screening, and show sharply contrasting trends in both incidence and mortality since the mid-1960s. Nearly complete coverage of the target population by organized cervical screening programmes in Iceland, Finland, Sweden, and parts of Denmark was soon followed by sharp falls in both incidence and mortality. In Norway, however, where an organized programme was not introduced, risk continued to increase up to the late 1970s.

Screening in the UK

With the exception of the North-East of Scotland, where a case–control study of cervical screening has shown a high relative protection from invasive cervical cancer in the first two years after a negative test, screening in Britain has been largely ineffective. There has only been a modest reduction in the overall incidence of invasive cervical cancer. This is mainly because screening has so far failed to reach the population who are most at risk of developing invasive cervical cancer. At least two-thirds of invasive cancer patients have never been screened at all. In the past in as many as 15 per cent of cases of invasive cancer there has been a failure to ensure adequate follow-up of an abnormal smear. Also in many cases, the interval between screens has been greater than 5 years.

Following Department of Health guidelines in January 1988, the aim is to reduce mortality from cervical cancer by regularly screening all eligible women in order to identify and treat conditions that might otherwise develop into cancer (Health Circular HC (88) 1) (DHSS 1988).

Trends in incidence

Trends in the UK between 1971 and 1984 show that there has been a significant increase in the incidence of both carcinoma *in situ* and invasive carcinoma for **young women**. Between 1971 and 1984 in the age-group 25–34 years the rates have more than doubled for invasive carcinoma and have trebled for carcinoma *in situ*. Carcinoma *in situ* and severe dysplasia are now considered together as cervical

Which is it in situ in vasive

intraepithelial neoplasia grade 3 (CIN 3). For carcinoma *in situ* there has been little change in the rates in other age-groups, but for invasive carcinoma the rates have decreased in the older age-groups, particularly for women aged 45–54 years.

These trends need however to be carefully interpreted, because they are influenced by the increase in screening, particularly in younger women. Thus at least part of the trend in age-specific incidence may be the result of the screening programme and not a true increase, though there is certainly a true increase in mortality in younger women.

Number of smears taken

The total number of cervical smear tests carried out by the NHS in England and Wales during 1987/8 was 4 322 000, as compared with 2 545 000 in 1977. The number of smears taken has increased by 11 per cent since 1986, and 70 per cent since 1977. It is uncertain to what extent this reflects an increase in screening activity, as these figures include both smears taken from symptomatic women and follow-up of women with previous abnormal smears. The 4.3 million smears currently being taken annually would be sufficient to screen all women aged 20 to 64 at a 5-year interval.

Abnormal smears

Some 43 052 (1 per cent) of the smears taken in 1987/8 were 'abnormal'. The number of abnormal results has increased by 16 per cent since 1986 and by 188 per cent since 1977.

The increased rate of abnormal smears may reflect:

- A possible increase in the disease.
- An increase in screening activity.
- An increase in diagnosis reflecting less stringent diagnostic criteria for 'abnormal' smears in recent years.

Information on abnormal smears is difficult to interpret, as the natural history of the disease is not well understood. The age of women with abnormal smears shows a significantly younger distribution than that for cases of invasive disease. However, it must be emphasized that smears taken are not representative of the whole population, but only of women who have been screened; and younger women are more likely to have been screened.

Natural history and frequency of screening

There is still considerable uncertainty about the natural history of the disease following an abnormal smear. There is a large discrepancy between the incidence of abnormal smears and the incidence of invasive cancer in unscreened women. This is because the majority of these 'abnormal' lesions will revert to normal spontaneously. Thus not all women with abnormal smears will go on to develop invasive disease. Others, however, may develop rapidly growing cancers. Even with an efficient cervical screening service, it is inevitable that an occasional case will be missed.

Because the natural history is not well understood, the optimum interval for screening remains a subject of debate. The evidence suggests that it is more important to provide effective coverage of the whole target age-range than to reduce the interval between screening (see p. 57).

Age

Although the observed increase in incidence in younger women may be attributable in part to the screening programme, it is widely believed that there has been a true rise in incidence in pre-invasive and invasive disease in the last 15 years in women under 35.

Despite this, it is **not** in fact younger women who are at the highest risk. More than half the smears are being taken from women under the age of 35, among whom only 16 per cent of cases of invasive cancer occur. This situation has evolved largely because of opportunistic screening in connection with family planning and maternity services. Overfrequent screening of younger women will produce numerous 'abnormals', many of which would probably regress. Investigation frequently causes undue anxiety, and has little effect on the overall morbidity or mortality from the disease. This uneven distribution of resources seems distorted when one considers that 84 per cent of invasive disease occurs in women aged 35 and over, the vast majority of whom have never been screened. To be most effective screening must concentrate on a wide age-range, with every effort being made to reach those at relatively higher risk of developing invasive cancer, namely older women of lower social class.

Mortality

In 1988, 2170 women died of cervical cancer in the UK (see Fig. 3). Ninety-four per cent of these cases were in women

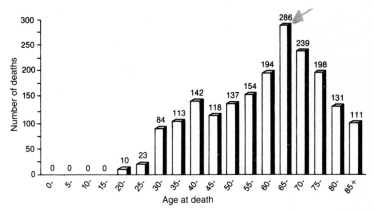

Fig. 3. Invasive cancer of the cervix—deaths, England and Wales, 1988. (Source: Factsheet 12, 1990.)

aged 35 and over. Over the last 20 to 30 years there has been a marked decrease in the mortality of women aged 45 and over (see Fig. 4). Since 1970 rates in women aged 50 to 59 have fallen from 20 to 10 deaths per 100 000. Moreover, the rise in deaths in women aged 40 to 44, observed in the late 1970s and 1980s, has now reversed. For women under 40 a significant increase in mortality was observed in the 1970s and 1980s. However, rates in this age group now appear to be stabilizing (see Fig. 4). The reversal of earlier trends which is now apparent may be due to an increase in screening over the past decade.

It should be noted that the number of deaths from cervical

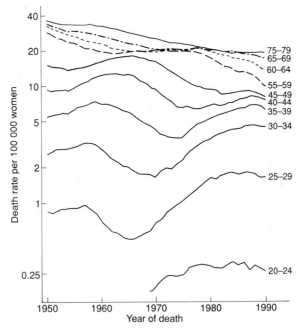

Fig. 4.   Age specific death rates for cervical cancer, England and Wales, 1950–90. (Source: Sasieni, 1991.)

cancer in women under the age of 35 remains comparatively small (about 110 deaths per annum) in relation to the total number of deaths from cervical cancer.

There is a considerable regional variation in cervical cancer mortality in the UK, showing a marked North–South divide. Analysis of the figures for DHAs show that the 20 DHAs with the highest standardized mortality ratios are all in the northern half of the country.

4   The call–recall system

Organization

Organization of cervical screening will vary from one Health Authority to another and from one practice to another. The call–recall system can be administered either by the local Health Authority or Family Health Services Authority (FHSA) or from within the practice itself. Whatever the case, it is important to run an efficient system and to have good co-operation with the programme manager who co-ordinates the local screening programme.

Suggestions are given in the following chapters which we hope practices will find useful. There is no single **right** method. Rather the best procedure will depend on the type of practice, the type and stability of the population, the staff employed, and the interests of the doctors and nurses.

Identify someone to organize cervical screening: Identify one person who will have overall responsibility (this can be the nurse, doctor, practice manager, receptionist, etc.).

Give the practice team the facts: Ensure that everybody in the practice understands their role in order to offer an effective screening programme (see Chapter 5).

The call-recall system in the practice: a protocol

A protocol for a call-recall system in the practice is shown in Fig. 5. Each aspect will be dealt with separately in subsequent chapters.

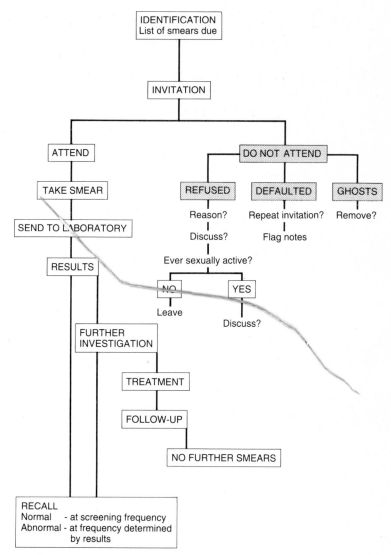

Fig. 5.   The practice cervical screening call–recall system.

5 The role of the primary care team in cervical screening

Primary care cervical screening activities are summarized in Table 2.

Table 2. Cervical screening—primary care activities

- Setting up and running a systematic screening programme
- Ensuring coverage of the target population
- Following up women who did not respond to the invitation
- Taking cervical smears
- Communicating with the laboratory
- Dealing with normal smear results
- Dealing with 'not normal' smear results
- Minimizing patient anxiety and dissatisfaction
- Running an effective fail-safe system
- Monitoring and evaluating the screening programme

Everyone in the practice team has a part to play in ensuring that women know they need regular cervical smears, making sure that they have the smear taken, and that they are informed of their results. Suggestions follow; but, of course, not all these people are needed in a practice to enable it to offer an effective screening programme:

Practice manager or secretary:

- Helps to set up the administration system within the practice.
- Communicates with the FHSA.

Doctor:

- Gives someone the responsibility of organizing the pro-gramme.
- Remembers to talk to patients about smears when they are seen in surgery for other problems.
- Checks on the cervical screening status of all new patients and patients not seen for three years.
- Takes the smears or arranges for the nurse or midwife to take them.
- Discusses screening with non-attenders either directly or on an opportunistic basis.

Practice nurse:

- Checks the cervical screening status of patients seen at the initial health check or 3-yearly check or when seen opportunistically.
- Takes the smears or arranges for them to be taken.
- Arranges to go on a special training course to learn tech-nique (if not done previously).
- Discusses screening with non-attenders either directly or on an opportunistic basis.

Receptionist:

- Puts up a notice in the waiting-room saying: 'Are you up to date with your cervical smear?'
- Checks leaflets are available.
- Checks patients' address details.
- Reminds the doctor or nurse of women coming to that day's surgery who need smears, or who have not attended for their smear.

Health visitor:

- Discusses cervical smear with patients and others in the houses visited.
- Supplies leaflets.

District nurse:

- Discusses screening with women in the correct age-group.

Midwife:

- Discusses screening with women in the antenatal and postnatal periods.
- Takes or arranges for smears to be taken, as appropriate.

6   Identification of women

Identification of eligible women

The FHSA will issue lists on a regular basis to all practices of women aged 20 to 64 who should be screened. Check the FHSA list against the practice list.

Identification of women who have never had a smear

Remember complete coverage of a wide age-range of women is essential if cervical screening is to be successful.

Most often the women who do not attend for screening are those at highest risk.

Two ways of achieving identification are:

Review the whole population of the practice: Send letters to women who have never had a smear, including an explanatory leaflet. Women who do not reply to an invitation can be approached again. If they still do not attend, mark this in their notes and either use the 'opportunistic' approach or approach them directly.

The 'opportunistic' approach: In this approach the practice receptionist plays a key role. The notes of defaulters should be flagged. The opportunity can be taken when a woman makes contact with the health centre or surgery not only to deal with the problem that has brought her there, but also to ask her if she would like a cervical smear test and to give her an explanatory leaflet. The opportunistic approach is useful as a back-up to a call system, as 75 per cent of women consult their GP in any one year and 90 per cent over a five-year period.

Some women may want to have the smear done at once if it can be arranged, thus avoiding a return visit; but for others it is better to make an appointment at a later, more convenient date. For women who have never had a smear, it may be best to try to do it then and there.

New patients

In accordance with the 1990 contract GPs should, where appropriate, seek details from newly registered patients or patients not seen within 3 years about cervical screening tests.

If the woman has had a smear before, immediately enter this into the recall system and tell her when her next smear is due.

If the woman needs a smear, do one, or arrange an appointment immediately and enter her into the appropriate recall system.

Temporary residents

Remember this group of women who may 'slip through the net' and never get asked about a cervical smear. They are not on an operative recall list because they move around a lot.

7   Invitation

Invitation letters

Letters of invitation can be sent from the FHSA or, if you prefer, you can use your own. The letter should be clear, short, and to the point. The following factors need to be taken into account when sending the letter of invitation:

- The purpose of the test should be clearly stated.
- The applicability of the test to the women should be stated, i.e. the letter should answer the question 'Why me?'

- A fixed appointment should if possible be given. This results in better uptake rates than asking the patient to make her own appointment.
- A reply slip helps practice organization.
- The availability of a woman doctor or nurse to take smear tests should be mentioned.
- A statement should be made on how results will be communicated.
- The letter should if possible be signed by a doctor whom the woman knows.
- A leaflet should be included.

8   Follow-up of non-attenders

Non-attenders fall into three categories: those who refuse to be screened, those who default, and 'ghosts'.

The practice can help to ensure that women receive an invitation by carefully checking the lists, and can play a part in educating women about the benefits and risks of cervical screening tests.

Refused smears: If a woman refuses to be screened, check if possible whether she has ever been sexually active. If she has, you may wish to discuss screening further with her in order to understand her attitudes and beliefs. However, it is the woman's right to decide how to respond. She should be provided with accurate information to help her arrive at an informed decision. It is important not to create feelings of guilt or inadequacy.

Defaulted: Check that the address details are correct. Send out a second invitation letter. If the woman still defaults, highlight her notes with an external marker and record the fact that she did not attend in the notes. Discuss cervical screening next time she attends or contact her directly and offer to discuss screening with her.

Ghosts: Patients identified as ghosts should be removed from the list and FHSAs should be notified accordingly. This may be particularly relevant when calculating whether you have reached the target (see pp. 50–3).

9   Taking cervical smears

Taking a smear

The objective of taking a smear is to identify women whose cytological pattern is suggestive of CIN. One of the key factors determining the effectiveness of a cervical screening programme is the quality of smear-taking. Poor smear-taking can miss 20 per cent or more of pre-cancerous abnormalities in the cervix (BSCC 1989).

The smear itself is taken by scraping cells from the cervix at the junction between the endocervix (covered by columnar epithelium) and the ectocervix (covered by squamous epithelium). The anatomical position of the transformation zone varies. It is thought that the initial changes in carcinogenesis take place here, and therefore it is important to get cells from both the endo- and the ecto-cervix.

Choice of spatula

Primary screening should be carried out with an Aylesbury spatula, which has a tip which is longer than the Ayres spatula and is thought to be more likely to sample endo-cervical cells as well as transformation zone squamous cells. The flatter reverse end may be used for a patulous cervix or a vault smear.

Cytobrush

A cytobrush is used to sample the endocervix, and is mainly used in colposcopy clinics or when the cervix is distorted by surgery or local ablation. It may be used in addition to a spatula in some instances, for example when the woman has had two previous smears showing insufficient cells. Beware, as one is likely to get more bleeding; so get the spatula sample first. The cytobrush is *not* the method of choice in primary screening, because it does not always sample the transformation zone, and provides smears of sparse cellularity, which dry quickly and need very rapid fixation.

After taking a smear

Make sure that each woman knows the possible outcomes of having had a smear taken and the likelihood of the smear being abnormal. It may be helpful to give an explanatory leaflet.

Make sure that each woman knows when to expect her results and how she will receive them.

Adequate smears

Between 5 and 10 per cent of all smears are inadequate.

Taking adequate smears will remove the anxiety induced when women are asked to return for the repeat of inadequate smears and reduce the overall workload for practices. Also, in terms of the GP contract, the calculations of targets are based on adequate smear tests only.

A cervical smear if properly taken should contain cells from the whole of the transformation zone, which should therefore be adequately sampled (BSCC, 1989). Squamous epithelial cells will normally be the most numerous cell type. The main evidence of an adequate smear is that it should contain a sufficient quantity of epithelial cells, taking into account a woman's age and her hormonal status. Properly taken cervical smears are more likely to be achieved in the right surroundings, i.e. with privacy, good lighting, and a comfortable woman.

An indication that the transformation zone has been properly sampled is the additional presence of endocervical columnar cells and recognizable metaplastic cells. Owing to the variable nature of the transformation zone *only one* of these cell types may be present on the smear. Endocervical cells may not always be seen in smears from post-menopausal women or those with atrophic smears.

Adequate smears and endocervical cells

- The main evidence of an adequate smear is a sufficient quantity of epithelial cells.

- Endocervical cells do *not* necessarily have to be present for the smear to be adequate, and, unless otherwise advised, the next smear should be carried out at the normal screening interval.

If a smear is inadequate the woman will need to have it repeated. She should be informed why the repeat smear is required, so as to allay the anxiety that this is likely to cause her.

Some reasons why smears may be reported as inadequate are given in Table 3.

Table 3.   Reasons for failure of the cervical smear test

- Patient very tense owing to failure of reassurance.
- Cervix not visualized adequately.
- Cervix not scraped firmly enough.
- Transformation zone not completely scraped.
- Material incompletely transferred to the slide.
- Sample poorly spread (too thick or too thin or distortion due to excessive pressure).
- Smear allowed to dry before fixation.
- Insufficient fixative used.
- Smear consisting mainly of blood or inflammatory cell exudate, possibly associated with menstruation.
- Contamination of the smear with lubricant, vaginal cream, or spermicide.
- Menstrual smears containing large numbers of endometrial cells.

Source: BSCC (1989). *Taking cervical smears*, p. 17.
The BSCC information booklet describes very clearly how these problems can be overcome.

Training

General practitioners and practice nurses have a central role in ensuring the quality of smears. Training courses for practice nurses should be provided locally, and practice nurses should be encouraged to attend.

Both the British Society for Clinical Cytology (BSCC) and the English National Board (ENB) have produced excellent videos on taking cervical smears (see *Resources* for details on how to obtain these). The BSCC booklet which accompanies the video provides very clear photographs of a wide range of cervical appearances.

10 Communicating with the laboratory

Good communication with your local cytology laboratory is a prerequisite for a successful cervical screening programme.

The Cervical Cytology Form is the basis of accurate cytology records. Accurate and complete records are essential to ensure:

- Accurate matching in the laboratory of:

    Current request form and slide for examination.
    Present request with previous smear history.

- The matching of smear results with FHSA records.

(Copies of the results must be sent to the sender of the

smear and to the GP (if not the same) unless the patient asks for them not to be.)

- The provision of clinical information to support the cytological diagnosis.

Demographic details: These are essential to make an accurate match between present and previous records and FHSA records. In descending order of importance they are:

> Name—first, second, and previous
> Date of birth
> NHS number
> Address

Clinical details: These are important for:

> Assessing the degree of urgency of the smear test.
> Supporting the cytological diagnosis.
> Enabling accurate assessment of normal findings.

Practical tip

In many practices, receptionists keep a record in a notebook of the names of women whose smears have been sent to the laboratory, and mark off when the results come back. It saves a lot of time should a woman ring up for her result.

---

11 Interpretation of the smear results

General

The appearance that is noted when cells are scraped from the surface of CIN lesions is called 'dyskaryosis'. Cytological reports of dyskaryosis are usually classified as mild, moderate, or severe.

It must be borne in mind that there is a whole spectrum of abnormality, from completely normal to definitely malignant, and cytological grading is an inexact science. Also the exact risk consequent on each grade is not clear.

It needs also to be remembered, when recommending further action, that referral of *all* grades of abnormality would lead to considerable over-investigation and over-diagnosis. A careful balance thus has to be reached, taking into account both the benefits that are likely to ensue and the costs, both to women and to the health service in terms of the resource implications. Inevitably opinions will differ on how such a balance is arrived at.

Smear results can sometimes be difficult to interpret. The smear may be normal in that there is no nuclear abnormality, but other comments may also be made about the smear. When a smear is reported with some abnormal cells, the action required will depend on many factors, including the appearance of any previous smears. If you do not understand a smear result, contact your local cyto-pathologist for clarification.

Normal smears

Smears should be coded as 'Negative' if there is no nuclear abnormality, in which case a repeat smear will *not* be necessary unless there is a history of previous abnormal smears or CIN (see Tables 4 and 5).

Other terminology may be used in describing smears which are negative (see Table 6). In some cases these may require other action by the GP, for example in the case of specific infections such as *Candida* or *Actinomyces*–like organisms. As long as there is no nuclear abnormality a repeat smear will not be necessary. Routine recall should be recommended.

Abnormal smears

All abnormal cervical smears should be assigned a result code depending on the degree of nuclear abnormality (see Table 5).

Borderline or mild dyskaryosis: One borderline or mildly dyskaryotic smear should be managed by a repeat smear at 6 months and consideration should be given to colposcopic referral if this is still not normal.

A minimum of two consecutive negative smears at least 6 months apart are needed before return to normal screening frequency (preferably 3-yearly).

Moderate dyskaryosis: Refer for colposcopy.

Severe dyskaryosis: Refer for colposcopy.

Invasive carcinoma/glandular neoplasia: Refer for colposcopy.

In practice it has been found in many instances that mild and moderate dyskaryotic smears do not correlate well with the histological diagnosis of mild or moderate dysplasia, i.e. CIN 1 or CIN 2. The difference is more in the quantity of CIN rather than the quality. CIN 3 in the presence of mild or moderate dyskaryosis generally speaking occupies a smaller proportion of the transformation zone than when it exists in the presence of severe dyskaryosis on the smear. Women with one moderately dyskaryotic or two mildly dyskaryotic smears should be referred for colposcopy. One can expect to find a fairly large proportion of CIN 3 in such women.

What proportion of screened women have abnormal smears?

Borderline or mild dyskaryosis—4 to 5 per cent of all smears.

Moderate or severe dyskaryosis—1.5 to 2.0 per cent of all smears.

Inadequate—5 to 10 per cent of all smears.

Wart virus infection

Wart virus or human papilloma virus (HPV) infection is suggested by koilocytosis, individual cell keratinization, and binucleation.

In practice it may be difficult to differentiate between subclinical HPV without CIN 1 and subclinical HPV with CIN 1 by cytology, colposcopy, or histology; but histological criteria do exist for distinguishing between CIN 1, sub-clinical HPV, and mixed lesions.

Cell changes suggesting infection with HPV are no longer in themselves considered an indication for more frequent screening if there is no nuclear atypia. However the majority of smears showing evidence of HPV will also have nuclear abnormalities. Such smears should be managed according to the CIN grade present and not simply the presence of HPV.

Changes suggesting HPV infection *without* nuclear change are rare. These should be coded 'Negative' and will not, therefore, indicate the need for more frequent follow-up. The presence of a viral change should *not* be recorded if it will not alter the management of the woman (i.e. if it is not accompanied by nuclear changes).

Table 4.   Interpretation of smears: summary of recommendations

---

- A smear showing borderline nuclear mildly dyskaryotic change should be repeated 6 months later and consideration should be given to colposcopic referral only if it is not then normal.

- A minimum of 2 consecutive negative smears at least 6 months apart are needed following a borderline or mildly dyskaryotic smear before surveillance is reduced to the normal screening frequency (preferably 3-yearly).

- Moderate and severe dyskaryosis should be referred for colposcopy straight away.

- Management of women with HPV must be according to the CIN grade present and not simply because of the presence of HPV.

- Smears showing viral change but no nuclear change should be considered normal, and the women should be recalled at normal frequency.

Source: I. Duncan (ed.), *Draft guidelines for clinical practice and programme management* (NHSCSP 1991).

Table 5.   Interpretation of smear results: result codes and action

Result code	Explanation	Action
Inadequate	Insufficient cellular material Inadequate fixation Smear consisting mainly of blood or inflammatory cell exudate Little or no material to suggest that the transformation zone has been sampled	Repeat smear
Negative	Normal. Includes simple inflammatory changes including a mild polymorph exudate.	Routine recall
Borderline changes, with or without HPV change	Cellular appearances that cannot be described as normal. Smears in which there is doubt as to whether the nuclear changes are inflammatory or dyskaryosis	Repeat smear at 6 months. Consider for colposcopy if changes persist.
Mild dyskaryosis with or without HPV change	Cellular appearances consistent with origin from CIN 1 (mild dysplasia)	Repeat smear at 6 months. Consider for colposcopy if changes persist.

Moderate dyskaryosis with or without HPV change	Cellular appearances consistent with origin from CIN 2 (moderate dysplasia)	Refer for colposcopy.
Severe dyskaryosis with or without HPV change	Cellular appearances consistent with origin from CIN 3 (severe dysplasia/carcinoma *in situ*)	Refer for colposcopy.
Severe dyskaryosis/ ? invasive carcinoma	Cellular appearances consistent with origin from CIN 3, but with additional features which suggest the possibility of invasive cancer	Refer for colposcopy.
Glandular neoplasia or suspicion of glandular neoplasia	Cellular appearances suggesting pre-cancer or cancer in the cervical canal or the endometrium	Refer for colposcopy.

Sources: BSCC, *Taking cervical smears*, 1989, p. 18; A. McPherson, *Cervical screening: a practical guide* (first edition), (OUP, 1985); I. Duncan (ed.), *Draft guidelines for clinical practice and programme management* (NHSCSP, 1991).
Note: The use of the term 'atypical cells' is no longer recommended in the Result Codes and its use should be discontinued. The preferred term is 'Borderline changes' ('atypia' may still be used in the free-text comment, but the degree of atypia should be clarified in the Result Code).

Table 6.   Interpretation of specific negative cervical smear reports

Result code	Explanation	Action
Specific infections	*Trichomonas, Candida* and cell changes associated with *Herpes simplex* can be identified	*Trichomonas*–treat *Candida*–treat if symptoms *Herpes*–no treatment–discuss with patient
Actinomyces	Organisms associated with IUD	No consensus. Alternatives: 1. Do nothing unless other symptoms e.g. pain or discharge 2. Change coil and the actinomyces organisms will disappear
Endocervical cells	Cells from the glandular epithelium of the cervical canal. During its formation the transformation zone will include similar epithelium	No action needed
Metaplastic cells (metaplasia/ squamous metaplasia)	Normal cells from the transformation zone	No action needed

Cytolysis	Normal process of cell disintegration	No action needed
Endometrial cells	Cells derived from the endometrial lining of the uterine cavity. Shed during menstruation and in some other circumstances	If IUD present–probably normal finding. If 1–12 day of 28 day cycle–normal finding. Otherwise discuss with laboratory or local gynaecologist.
Inflammatory changes	Cellular appearance present in some degree in many smears and not evidence of CIN	No consensus. Alternatives: 1. Do nothing 2. Take high vaginal swabs for culture and sensitivity and take chlamydial swabs. Then treat as necessary
Atrophic smear	Common in postmenopausal smears, i.e. when oestrogen and progesterone levels are low. Similar changes are seen in postnatal smears	No action needed

Result codes

Although it will not always be possible to standardize the free-text comments which a cytologist reports on the form, the Result, Infection, and Action Codes should be standardized and consistent with each other. If this is not the case, seek clarification from your cytopathologist. Some specific examples are given below:

1. HPV should *not* be recorded with a 'Negative' Result Code. Those changes that are regarded as sufficiently abnormal to warrant an early repeat smear should be coded as 'Borderline' or 'Mild Dyskaryosis'. Otherwise they need not and should not be recorded.

2. Severe inflammation should not be accompanied by a 'Negative' Result Code. A decision should be made as to whether the smear was unsatisfactory for screening (an 'Inadequate' Result) or whether there was doubt as to the presence or absence of dyskaryosis (a 'Borderline' Result).

3. Infections such as *Candida*, *Herpes*, *Actinomyces*, and some cases of follicular cervicitus may be recorded for information and may be combined with a 'Negative' Result Code and the recommendation for routine screening. If the cellular changes or degree of exudate warrant early follow-up, then the Result Code should be recorded as 'Inadequate' or 'Borderline'.

12 Giving results

Giving results to women with normal smears

It is important that women are given the results of their smear. This can be done by:

- Asking women to phone in for the result. This transfers the responsibility from the practice to the woman and is neither satisfactory nor efficient. Also staff need to be cautious about giving results over the telephone. If you do it this way, make sure it is recorded properly.
- Writing to women. This is the recommended procedure and a standard letter can be used.

An example of such a letter is shown below:

Example of normal results letter to patients

Dear

I now have the result of your recent cervical smear which I am pleased to say was normal.

Our present policy is that you should have a smear every .... years: we will, therefore, recall you in .... years' time.

If you have any symptoms that worry you, please don't hesitate to contact me earlier.

Yours sincerely,

Dr ....

Record in the woman's notes that the result has been given.

- There are in addition systems which can produce a computer printout to be sent directly from the laboratory to the woman, with a copy going to the GP. This is often the most efficient and expeditious way of issuing results.

Giving results to women with abnormal smears

The way in which a patient is told about an abnormal smear will often affect how she will cope with any treatment or future follow-up. Unfortunately there is no 'ideal' way, and many women told they have an abnormality in their smear may panic, or at least will want to have more information. Advising women at the time of smear-taking about the possibility of an abnormal smear result sometimes helps.

According to recent research, information and support are needed particularly in the following areas, to avoid unnecessary anxiety:

Informing women of the result: The most effective and efficient way of conveying this is to ensure that each woman receives her result in writing. It is essential to ensure that the information is understandable and not alarming. Women who need a referral to colposcopy or who have invasive disease should be offered an early appointment or opportunity to speak with the GP to discuss the implications of the results. Waiting and uncertainty are often the most difficult part of the referral process. Women with results requiring repeat smears at a shorter interval may also appreciate the opportunity to discuss this with their GP.

Some doctors will prefer to write a personalized letter to all patients who do not have a normal smear. Others use a standard format, as shown below, for patients requiring a repeat smear, and write personalized letters only to those requiring gynaecological referral. Sending an explanatory leaflet will also help. Whichever method is used, the woman needs to know the results quickly, and what the implications are for her. Record in the notes that the result has been communicated.

Example of an abnormal results letter to a patient requiring a repeat smear

Dear

Your cervical smear shows a slightly abnormal cellular pattern, but there is no cause for concern and no treatment required. You are advised to have another smear in .... months' time. An appointment will be sent to you nearer the time. If you want any additional information please do not hesitate to come and see me.

Yours sincerely,

Dr ....

Explaining the meaning of an abnormal smear: If the result is not normal it is often assumed that it means cancer. It is therefore important to explain exactly what the abnormality is, what you think it is due to, and what further steps in investigation, follow up, and treatment may be needed. Explaining terms, for example 'dyskaryosis', 'CIN', and 'pre-invasive cancer', is important.

Explaining investigation and treatment: Many women do not know what will be involved when they are referred for colposcopy, and will need information about the nature of the procedure. Also explain possible treatments, such as excision biopsy, destructive treatment, or hysterectomy, before a woman is referred. Depending on age, many will want to know how the treatment will affect their sex lives and their chances of future pregnancies.

Giving practical advice: Give information about intercourse, future contraception, pregnancy, and the use of tampons, as patients may feel inhibited about discussing these issues.

Arranging future follow-up: Always consider inviting the patient for future follow-up by the GP after she has attended the hospital, as this can be very reassuring.

Giving results to women with wart virus changes

Reporting of wart virus changes due to HPV in cervical smears poses particular problems, both for women and for smear-takers who have to explain the significance of any findings. Current lack of certainty about the role of the virus in the evolution of cervical cancer adds to the difficulty. Research suggests that the virus may be present in many women without any clinical or cytological manifestation.

The consensus view at present is that the management of women with HPV must be according to the CIN grade present, and not simply because the presence of HPV. Smears showing viral change but no nuclear change should be considered normal, and the woman should be recalled at normal frequency. The presence of a viral change should *not* be recorded if it will not alter the management of the woman.

If the presence of HPV is reported, women will need to know that:*

*Source: Oxfordshire DHA (1991). *Cervical screening information factsheet.*

- The wart virus in its subclinical state requires no specific treatment such as antibiotics. Referral to an STD/GUM clinic is not necessary.

- The changes are evidence of contact with the virus at some stage in the woman's life, and may not indicate an active infection.

- There are parallels with skin warts and many other viral conditions, where only very few contacts develop the clinical infection.

- The virus is usually transmitted sexually; but this is *not* the only way, as it has been isolated from other sites in the body and has also been found in children.

- The natural history of wart virus changes is to regress over a period of several years. One particular strain of the virus, HPV16, may be an important prognostic marker for identifying patients who are at risk of developing severe cervical disease. Other factors such as smoking or lowered immunity may also come into play.

- In a steady relationship there is no need to change contraception; but if a woman is likely to have any sexual contact outside an established relationship, barrier methods might be used.

- Subclinical warts are not known to affect pregnancy, fertility, or the baby. Clinical warts should be treated prior to delivery.

- Visible cervical warts are thought to be more easily transmitted than subclinical HPV. Patients do not necessarily need to be referred to an STD/GUM clinic, and should encourage their partners to be examined.

NOTE: Colposcopic treatment does not eradicate the presence of wart virus.

13 Colposcopy

What is colposcopy?

The colposcope is a low-powered microscope for viewing the cervix. During the investigation the patient lies on her back with her legs up in stirrups. A speculum is passed into the vagina to visualize the cervix before using the colposcope. The colposcope is mainly used for the investigation and management of cervical intra-epithelial neoplasia (CIN).

Colposcopy is performed by specially trained clinicians. It takes about 15 minutes to carry out, and should not be painful, although it can cause short-lived discomfort. It allows the clinician to view the cervix very carefully in order to assess the extent and severity of any lesion properly and to provide appropriate treatment. A sample of tissue can be taken from the cervix if necessary.

Who needs colposcopy?

CIN may be suspected in patients with abnormal cervical cytology; but diagnosis and treatment will depend upon referral of such women for colposcopic assessment.

The two main indications for colposcopy are:

1. To investigate an abnormal smear (see Table 5). It can be combined with endocervical curettage and punch biopsy if necessary.
2. For more thorough assessment of a clinically suspicious cervix, even in the presence of a normal smear.

Moderate and severe dyskaryosis should be an indication for colposcopy. A borderline or mildly dyskaryotic smear should be managed by a repeat smear at six months, with referral for colposcopy only if the abnormality persists. In occasional cases an earlier repeat may be requested. Referrals for colposcopy should be based on the degree of dyskaryosis, with the exception of the clinically suspicious cervix, which should indicate referral to a gynaecologist for appropriate investigation and biopsy regardless of the smear result.

What proportion of women require colposcopy?

Approximately 2 to 4 per cent of all smears will be referred for colposcopy, depending on how often smears showing minor abnormalities are repeated before referral.

Results from a colposcopy clinic in Dundee show the following for colposcopic referral:

Table 7. Relative occurrence of reasons for referral to colposcopy

	Per cent of colposcopic referrals
Following 2 mildly dyskaryotic smears	40.5
Following 1 moderately dyskaryotic smear	44.5
Following 1 severely dyskaryotic smear	15.0

Information about colposcopy

Women undergoing colposcopy may experience very high levels of anxiety about both the procedure and the outcome. Research has shown that anxiety and distress is considerably less in women who, prior to the appointment for colposcopy, have the procedure explained to them, and who receive a leaflet detailing what could happen. They will also require information during and after the procedure.

14   Treatment

When should the cervix be treated?

In order to know when to treat the cervix, it is important to have some idea of the rate of progression of abnormalities. Those at high risk of progression must be treated. There is currently inadequate information about the natural history of the lower grades of abnormality. The majority may not progress, but some would lead eventually to invasive disease if not treated at any stage. A balance must thus be reached between potential over-diagnosis and over-treat-ment, and the need to ensure that progression to invasive cancer does not occur. It is therefore not possible to define a treatment policy with any degree of certainty. While CIN 1 falls at the low-risk end of the spectrum and CIN 3 at the high-risk end, CIN 2 is more difficult to categorize. On balance it is currently believed that CIN 2 should be treated in the same way as CIN 3. Those at low risk of progression can either be treated or managed by close observation.

At colposcopy samples can be taken from the cervix, and, if histological diagnosis indicates CIN 2 or 3, the affected part of the cervix is removed or destroyed. Women with CIN 1 may be treated or kept under close surveillance.

When should the cervix be treated?

- CIN 2 and CIN 3 should be treated once diagnosed
- CIN 1 may be treated or kept under close surveillance

General points about treatment

Extremes of heat or cold are essentially equally effective in killing cells in the transformation zone of the cervix. Laser ablation, 'cold' coagulation (which actually boils the cells), electrocoagulation diathermy, and cryosurgery are all in current use. Alternatively the transformation zone may be excised using a laser or a large cutting electrosurgical loop (Large Loop Excision of the Transformation Zone, LLETZ). Cervical function is not compromised.

In all instances the woman will experience uterine contractions, mainly of the intensity of menstrual cramps, but occasionally like labour pains. Local anaesthetic is only of limited value; but general anaesthetic is rarely required. In some circumstances where the whole of the transformation zone is not visible, or microinvasion or a significant glandular abnormality is suspected, or the patient has been previously treated, a cone biopsy may be required; and, even more rarely, a hysterectomy may be suggested. The method of management will depend on local preferences and facilities.

Some methods of treatment involve two visits; in others, for example large loop excision, diagnosis and treatment are dealt with in a single visit—which has obvious advantages for the patients.

Present methods of treatment

Local destructive therapy:
   Carbon-dioxide laser ablation
   'Cold' coagulation
   Electrocoagulation
   Diathermy
   Cryosurgery

Local excision:
   Knife cone biopsy (large cone)
   Laser cone biopsy (shallow cone)
   Large loop excision of the transformation zone (LLETZ)

Hysterectomy:
   (Rare)

15   Follow-up of treated patients

Reasons for follow-up

There are four reasons for follow-up:

- To identify residual disease
- To identify new CIN
- To identify new invasive disease
- To reassure both the patient and the clinician

The risks of the first three occurring are probably no different regardless of whether the patient has undergone an ablative or excisional technique.

How should follow-up be conducted?

Cytological follow-up is essential after treatment for CIN. Those patients who have undergone ablation or excision should be followed up cytologically. An endocervical brush may be needed if the cervix has healed with a very small aperture.

Colposcopy is not essential in the review process but may enhance detection of persistent disease.

Conservatively treated CIN 3

Cytological follow-up is essential.

Following treatment the first smear should be undertaken at 6 months, and, if normal, it should be repeated at 12 months.

Colposcopy may enhance detection of persistent disease at 6 months; but, if the findings are normal, further colposcopic assessment in the presence of normal cytology is not warranted.

If normal at 12 months, the patients should have yearly follow-up, and at 5 years should be returned to the normal screening frequency.

After hysterectomy

After hysterectomy the risks of residual or new disease are very low provided that the woman was colposcopically assessed prior to surgery to exclude occult disease at the top of the vagina.

Women who have had a hysterectomy for premalignancy should have persistent disease excluded by cytology at 6 and 12 months after surgery, and then no further smears if the cytology is normal.

Table 8.   Follow-up of treated patients: summary of recommendations

---

- Cytological follow-up is essential following treatment for CIN. Colposcopy is not essential, but may enhance detection of persistent disease at 6 months.

- Following treatment, the first smear should be taken at 6 months and, if normal, repeated at 12 months.

- More frequent surveillance need not be continued beyond 5 years of normal findings after conservative treatment for CIN 3.

- Women undergoing hysterectomy with a past or current history of CIN 3 need have no further smears if the cytology is normal 6 and 12 months after surgery.

Source: I. Duncan (ed.), *Draft guidelines for clinical practice and programme management* (NHSCSP 1991).

16 Running an effective fail-safe system

The responsibility of the general practitioner

The general practitioner has a key role in the fail-safe mechanism, contributing to it in several ways:

- Checking that all smear reports have been received
- Informing the woman of the result
- Initiating further investigation
- Contacting women who do not attend for further investigation
- Informing the FHSA if a woman requiring investigation has moved away
- Monitoring the 'suspend' and 'repeat advised' lists sent by the FHSA

Where smears are taken by GP trainees or practice nurses responsibility lies with the GP principal recorded on the request form.

Where smears are taken outside the primary-care setting and the result is sent to the GP, it is important to check who is looking after the follow-up and referral as necessary.

17 Funding issues: calculating targets

Since 1 April 1990, the item for service payments for cervical cytology has been replaced by quarterly target payments.

Currently payments will be triggered on reaching 50 per cent or 80 per cent coverage of the eligible population, with a differential of 3:1 in favour of the latter.

The eligible population and criteria for targets and claims

- Women aged 25–64
- Excluding only women who have had hysterectomies involving the complete removal of the cervix (there may be additional locally agreed criteria for exclusion)
- Smears taken in the 5.5 years preceding the claim
- Smears must have been 'adequate'

Calculation of coverage and payments

Coverage will be based on the list of a GP's patients as defined above, as calculated at the beginning of each quarter.

For the calculation of coverage, the smear can have been taken by *any* source, including private screening and family planning clinics.

Where either target is reached, *only* the proportion of adequate smears taken within the general medical services will be eligible for remuneration. Adequate smears taken by GPs for health authorities will not count towards the payment.

For payment purposes the number of eligible women on the GP's list will be compared with the number of eligible women on the list of the 'average' practitioner.

Where smears are repeated during the 5.5-year period, an adequate smear within the general medical services will take precedence over one from another service.

A protocol for calculating targets is shown in Fig. 6, and the relevant payment quarters are set out in Table 9.

Table 9.   Payment quarters

Quarter ending	Assessment date	Claim date
30 September	1st April	2nd August
30 December	1st July	2nd November
30 March	1st October	2nd February
30 June	1st January	2nd May

Calculating past coverage

Some FHSAs currently have inadequate data on smears taken over the 5 years prior to 1 April 1990. Interim arrangements may need to apply until April 1994, based on GP's own records. Options are:

● payment based on the practice's own computerized records. Criteria on the adequacy of records will need to be agreed with the FHSA, or

● practices will need to audit their own records using agreed guidelines. This will need a baseline audit of an

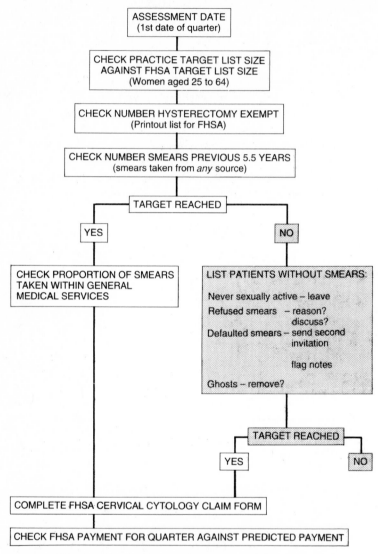

Fig. 6.   Cervical screening: target claim protocol.

agreed number of records, which can be extrapolated to the total eligible population and updated quarterly.

For both methods, where practice records do not show the adequacy of smears and the source of the smear, this data will need to be estimated from laboratory records or, if necessary, using FHSA averages.

Auditing 'inadequate' smears

It will be useful for practices to assess the number and percentage of inadequate smears. This can be done to cover a particular period of time, for example annually. Each practice will need to calculate:

- The total number of smears taken in the practice.
- The percentage inadequate for
  —the practice as a whole
  —individual takers.
- Comparison with the District as a whole.

NOTE: In auditing inadequate smears, the age profile of women should be taken into account, as inadequacy rate will be different in older and younger women.

Costs and time spent on cervical screening

It is useful in terms of the general management and overall audit of the practice to calculate the following:

- Time spent by administrative staff
- Percentage of smears done by the practice nurse
- Postage expenses (number of invitations and results sent out)

- Cost of stationery
- Cost of equipment/sterilization
- Training implications
- Cost of computerization

Targets: problems

Practices achieving:

    < 50 per cent—why bother?
                    —give up screening?
50-75 per cent—settle for 50 per cent and retain 'ghosts' rather than aim for 80 per cent?
   > 80 per cent—settle for 80 per cent and retain 'ghosts' rather than aim above this level?
75-79 per cent—use 'coercive' tactics to achieve 80 per cent?

18 Monitoring and evaluating the programme

In order to monitor and evaluate the effectiveness of the programme in the practice, the following information should be calculated on an annual basis:

- Coverage achieved
- Number of women invited
- Number of women screened
- Number of exclusions
- Age-range of women screened
- Number of inadequate smears
- Number of 'normal' smears
- Number of 'abnormal' smears in each category
- Number requiring repeat smears
- Number requiring colposcopy
- Number requiring treatment
- Number of refusers
- Number of defaulters

These should, where possible, be related to the overall results for the local screening programme.

19 Areas of uncertainty

Guidelines are currently being produced on a number of areas of cervical screening. This will allow for the development of a more consistent and uniform approach. However many areas still remain open to doubt and good research studies are required to resolve areas of controversy. Some of these issues are discussed below:

Is screening teenagers worthwhile?

The prevalence of invasive carcinoma of the cervix does not justify including women under the age of 20 in the routine screening programme provided that there is good uptake in women aged 20 to 25.

While CIN does exist in teenagers, invasive cancer is extremely rare. There is no rational basis for routinely screening teenagers, regardless of whether they are 'promiscuous' or not. Smears need not be taken in teenagers who have just become sexually active. This does not mean that a diagnostic test cannot be taken where a general practitioner thinks it is warranted in the individual case.

Is screening 65-year-olds and over worthwhile?

Although a substantial number of cases of cervical cancer occur in women aged 65 and over, an effective screening programme should detect precancerous lesions in those under 65, and thus reduce the incidence of invasive disease in older women. Women aged 65 and over should be encouraged to have a smear if they have not previously been screened.

How often should smears be taken?

The Department of Health has recommended that a smear should be taken 'at least every 5 years'. There is considerable local variation—some DHAs do 5-yearly screening, some 3-yearly, and some a mixture of both. This is further complicated by the fact that GP target payments relate to smears taken over a 5.5-year period.

Because the natural history of the disease is not well understood, the optimum interval remains a subject of debate and an important research issue. It has been estimated that if a woman is screened regularly from age 20 to 64 every 5 years, her risk of developing invasive disease would be reduced by 84 per cent. Decreasing the interval to 3 years would add 7 per cent protection, but would increase the number of smears taken in her lifetime from 9 to 15. Decreasing the interval further to 1 year between screens would add an additional 2 per cent protection, increasing the lifetime number of smears to 45 (Day, 1989).

Should high-risk women be screened more frequently?

Although there are several risk factors associated with an increased risk of invasive cervical cancer (see p. 5), it is *not* possible to use these factors to reliably predict which women will develop CIN. Moreover there is no evidence that these risk factors affect the rate of progression of CIN. There is thus little value in targeting these women for more frequent screening.

Should younger women be screened more frequently?

For younger women, particularly those aged 25 to 34, there has been a significant increase in cervical cancer incidence and mortality rates over the past 10 to 20 years. Some DHAs screen women under 35 years at 3-year intervals, and women of 35 years and over at 5-year intervals. There is no evidence to support this decision one way or another. Further research on the natural history of the disease is necessary, for example to clarify whether the disease is more aggressive in younger women or not.

Is there a role for cervicography?

Current studies of cervicography give a false-positive rate up to ten times higher than that for routine cervical smears, thereby leading to an unnecessarily high number of referrals for colposcopy. Cervicography may well pick up additional 'abnormalities', but the majority of these may be of no clinical significance. The cost of cervicography is much higher than that for the cervical smear.

Despite problems in the interpretation of cervical smears, cervicography cannot at present be seen as an alternative. There is currently no routine clinical role for cervicography in either primary cervical screening or in the further assessment of patients with abnormal cytology.

What is the appropriate management of mild dyskaryosis?

While the consensus view is that a single mildly dyskary-otic smear should be managed by a repeat smear at 6 months and only referred for colposcopy if the abnormality persists, there are those who believe that such smears should be referred immediately for colposcopy. This is because, while the majority of such smears will revert to normal or persist as mildly dyskaryotic, a small proportion may progress to severe dyskaryosis over a period of time. A balance obviously has to be achieved here between ensuring appropriate management and not subjecting too many women to unnecessary medical procedures. Further research is clearly needed to assess the role of cytological surveillance in mild dyskaryosis and to determine its optimal management. The Aberdeen Birthright Project has been set up to evaluate the safety and effectiveness of a cytology-based approach to the management of both mild and moderate dyskaryosis.

How should HPV be managed?

The role of HPV in cervical cancer causation is still uncertain. The apparent universal presence of the virus has been recognized, and adds to this uncertainty.

Cell changes suggesting HPV infection are no longer in themselves considered an indication for more frequent screening. *Management of women with HPV must be according to the CIN grade present, and not simply because of the presence of HPV. Smears showing viral change but no nuclear change should be considered normal and the woman recalled at normal frequency.*

The presence of a particular strain of the virus, HPV16, may be an important prognostic marker for identifying women who are at risk of developing severe cervical disease. At some time in the future, viral typing may be a second discriminator in the process of deciding which lesions to treat. This is not the case at present.

When should the cervix be treated?

There is a whole spectrum of abnormality from completely normal to definitely malignant. Ideally it is important to have some idea of the rate of progression of abnormalities. Currently, however, there is inadequate information available about the natural history of the lower grades of abnormality. A balance must thus be reached between potential overdiagnosis and overtreatment and the need to ensure that invasive cancer does not occur. A treatment policy cannot be defined with any degree of certainty. On balance the present belief is that CIN 2 and CIN 3 should be treated once diagnosed, while women with CIN 1 may be treated or kept under close surveillance.

Are targets a realistic way of improving uptake?

The introduction of targets has been very controversial. It *has* led to a marked increase in cervical screening activity, but raises many problems. Some of these were discussed on p. 54. An additional problem concerns the criteria for exclusion. Women who say 'no' cannot be excluded, and remain in the denominator of the target calculation. This creates a conflict, in that it goes against the spirit of enabling women to make informed choices about whether or not they wish to be screened.

References, Further reading

BSCC (1989). *Taking cervical smears*. British Society for Clinical Colposcopy, London.

Cancer Research Campaign Factsheets (1990). *Cervical cancer* (Factsheet 12), *Cervical cancer screening* (Factsheet 13).

Day, N. (1989). Screening for cancer of the cervix. *Journal of Epidemiology and Community Health*, **43**, 103–6.

DHSS (1988). *Health Circular HC (88)1*. Health Services Management, Cervical Cancer Screening.

DH (1988). *Cervical cytology and cervical cancer statistics 1976–1986, England and Wales.*

DH (1989). *Cervical cytology 1987/8.*

DH (1990). *Cervical cytology 1988/9.*

Duncan, I. (ed.) (1991). *Draft guidelines for clinical practice and programme management*. NHS Cervical Screening Programme, Oxford.

Eardley, A., Elkind, A., and Thompson, R. (1990). HEA guidelines for a letter to invite women for a smear test: theory and practice. *Health Education Journal*, **49**, 51–6.

Elkind, A., Eardley, A., Thompson, R., and Smith, A. (1990). *Operating cervical screening: The experience of District Health Authorities*. NHS Cervical Screening Programme, Oxford.

Havelock, C. M., Edwards, R., Cuzick, J., and Chamberlain, J. (1988). The organisation of cervical screening in general practice. *Journal of the Royal College of General Practitioners*, **38**, 207–11.

Oxfordshire DHA (1991). *Cervical Screening Information Factsheets*. Cytology Department, John Radcliffe Hospital, Oxford.

Posner, T. and Vessey, M. (1988). *Prevention of cervical cancer: the patient's view*. King Edward's Hospital Fund for London, London.

Quilliam, S. (1989). *Positive smear*. Penguin Books, London.

Sasieni, P. (1991). Trends in cervical cancer mortality. (Letter). *Lancet*, **338**, 818–9.

Singer, A. and Szarewski, A. (1988). *Cervical smear test*. Macdonald, London.

61

Wilkinson, C., Jones, J. M., and McBride, J. (1990). Anxiety caused by abnormal result of cervical smear test: a controlled trial. *British Medical Journal*, **300**, 440.

Wilson, A. and Leeming, A. (1987). Cervical cytology screening: a comparison of two call systems. *British Medical Journal*, **295**, 181–2.

Resources

BSCC Booklet and Video: *Taking cervical smears* (BSCC, 1989). For further information, contact:

Dr Keith Randall
Red Tree House
Pine Glade
Keston Park
ORPINGTON
Kent BR6 8NT

English National Board for Nursing—Video on Cervical Screening:

ENB
Resource and Careers Service
Woodseats House
764a Chesterfield Road
SHEFFIELD
Yorkshire S8 0SE

ICRF Video: *Cervical smears: the facts* (University of Oxford, 1987). For further information contact:

Department of Medical Illustration
University of Oxford
John Radcliffe Hospital
Headington
OXFORD OX3 9DU

Useful addresses

Cancer Research Campaign
2 Carlton House Terrace
LONDON SW1 5AR   Tel: 071 930 8972

Cancer Research Campaign Primary Care Education Group
University of Oxford
65 Banbury Road   Tel: 0865 310457
OXFORD OX2 6PE   Fax: 0865 58149

Health Education Authority (HEA)
Hamilton House
Mabledon Place
LONDON WC1H 9TX   Tel: 071 383 3833

Imperial Cancer Research Fund
Lincolns Inn Fields
P.O. Box 123
LONDON WC2A 3PX   Tel: 071 242 0200

Scottish Health Education Group
Woodburn House
Canaan Lane
EDINBURGH
Scotland   Tel: 031 447 8044

Tenovus Cancer Information Centre
11 Whitchurch Road
CARDIFF CF4 3JN
Wales   Tel: 0222 619846

Ulster Cancer Foundation
40–42 Eglantine Avenue
BELFAST BT9 6DX
Northern Ireland   Tel: 0232 663281/2/3

Women's National Cancer Control Campaign
1 South Audley Street
LONDON W1Y 5DQ   Tel: 071 499 7532/3/4

19   91
20 91
72
────────
19 29